NIA TECHNIQUE

FOR BEGINNERS

A Comprehensive Guide For Beginners To Enhance
Body-Mind Connection, Boost Flexibility, And
Improve Overall Well-Being

ROBERT LUGO

CHAPTER 1
Introduction To Nia Technique

The Nia technique is a holistic approach to fitness and well-being that integrates movement, mindfulness, and self-expression.

It offers a unique blend of dance, martial arts, and healing arts, creating a versatile and engaging practice suitable for people of all ages and fitness levels.

Understanding the core concepts of the Nia technique is essential for beginners embarking on this journey of self-discovery and physical empowerment.

What is the Nia Technique?

At its essence, the Nia technique is a dynamic fusion of dance, martial arts, and healing arts.

It was founded by Debbie Rosas and Carlos Rosas in the 1980s, to provide a joyful and transformative movement experience. Nia stands for "Neuromuscular Integrative Action," emphasizing the integration of body, mind, emotions, and spirit in movement.

Unlike traditional exercise programs, Nia encourages participants to explore their unique movement styles, fostering a sense of freedom and self-expression.

History and Origins of Nia

The history of the Nia technique traces back to the pioneering work of Debbie Rosas and Carlos Rosas. They drew inspiration from various movement modalities, including dance, yoga, martial arts, and Feldenkrais.

Their vision was to create a fitness practice that not only nourishes the body but also nurtures the soul.

Over the years, Nia has evolved into a global movement, with certified instructors and passionate practitioners across the world.

Central to the Nia philosophy are the principles of Joy of Movement, Awareness, and Body-Mind-Spirit Integration.

Joy of Movement celebrates the pleasure and playfulness of moving in ways that feel good to the body. Awareness invites participants to cultivate mindful attention to sensations, emotions, and thoughts during movement. Body-mind-spirit integration emphasizes the interconnectedness of physical, mental, and spiritual aspects of well-being, promoting holistic health and vitality.

Benefits of Practicing Nia

The benefits of practicing Nia are manifold and extend beyond physical fitness. On a physical level, Nia improves cardiovascular health, strength, flexibility, and agility. It also enhances coordination, balance, and posture, contributing to overall functional fitness. Beyond the physical benefits, Nia promotes emotional well-being by providing a creative outlet for self-expression and stress relief.

It fosters mental clarity, focus, and mindfulness, supporting holistic health and resilience.

Why Nia is Suitable for Beginners

Nia is highly suitable for beginners due to its inclusive and adaptable nature. Unlike traditional fitness programs that may focus solely on physical conditioning, Nia embraces a holistic approach that considers individual needs and preferences. Beginners can ease into Nia at their own pace, gradually exploring movement patterns and discovering their unique expressions. The non-competitive and non-judgmental environment of Nia classes encourages beginners to embrace their bodies and enjoy the journey of self-discovery and empowerment.

CHAPTER 2
Understanding Nia Movements

Nia, short for Neuromuscular Integrative Action, is a holistic fitness practice that combines dance, martial arts, and healing arts. At its core, Nia is about embodying movement with pleasure, mindfulness, and self-expression.

Understanding Nia movements involves delving into its three core principles, exploring the repertoire of 52 Nia Moves, and recognizing the deep mind-body connection it fosters.

The Three Core Principles of Nia: Dance, Martial Arts, Healing Arts

Nia's foundation lies in its three core principles: Dance, Martial Arts, and Healing Arts. Dance infuses Nia with expressive movement, fluidity, and grace, allowing practitioners to tap into their creative energy and individual style. Martial Arts brings elements of strength, precision, and mindfulness, incorporating techniques from Tai

Chi, Tae Kwon Do, and Aikido to cultivate power and agility. Healing Arts completes the trio by integrating principles of body awareness, relaxation, and self-healing, creating a nurturing environment for physical and emotional well-being. Together, these principles form a comprehensive approach to movement that is both dynamic and holistic.

Exploring the 52 Nia Moves

Central to Nia practice are the 52 Nia Moves, a diverse set of movements inspired by dance, martial arts, and everyday functional activities. These moves range from flowing gestures to dynamic strikes, from gentle stretches to powerful kicks, providing a rich vocabulary for self-expression and fitness enhancement.

Each move in the Nia repertoire is designed to target specific muscle groups, improve flexibility, enhance coordination, and stimulate overall body awareness. By exploring and mastering these moves, practitioners can unlock new levels of strength, agility, and joy in their movement practice.

Embodying Sensation and Pleasure in Movement

One of the unique aspects of Nia is its emphasis on sensation and pleasure in movement.

Unlike traditional fitness approaches that focus solely on physical exertion, Nia encourages practitioners to tune into their body's sensations, rhythms, and feedback. This mindful approach not only enhances the effectiveness of workouts but also fosters a deeper connection with one's body and emotions. By cultivating a sense of pleasure and enjoyment in movement, Nia promotes sustainable fitness habits and a positive relationship with exercise.

Mind-Body Connection in Nia

The mind-body connection is at the heart of Nia's philosophy.

Through mindful movement, breath awareness, and sensory exploration, practitioners learn to synchronize their physical actions with mental focus and emotional expression.

This integrated approach not only improves physical fitness but also nurtures mental clarity, emotional resilience, and stress reduction.

By cultivating a strong mind-body connection, Nia empowers individuals to move with intention, authenticity, and joy, both on and off the dance floor.

CHAPTER 3
Nia Technique Anatomy

Anatomy Basics for Nia Practitioners

Understanding anatomy is fundamental for practitioners of the Nia Technique, as it forms the basis for movement efficiency, body awareness, and overall well-being. Nia practitioners delve into the intricate details of human anatomy to enhance their understanding of how the body moves and functions. This knowledge empowers them to perform Nia movements with precision, grace, and safety.

In Nia, anatomy basics encompass a holistic view of the body, including bones, muscles, joints, and connective tissues. Practitioners learn about the skeletal structure and its role in providing support and mobility. They explore the muscular system, understanding how muscles work in pairs or groups to create movement and stability. Joint anatomy is also a crucial aspect, as it influences the range of motion and fluidity of movements in Nia routines.

Furthermore, Nia practitioners study the fascial network, which includes the fascia, tendons, and ligaments. This interconnected web of tissues plays a vital role in transmitting forces throughout the body, contributing to strength, flexibility, and coordination. By grasping the basics of anatomy, Nia practitioners gain insights into how to optimize their movements, prevent injuries, and promote overall physical health.

Body Awareness and Alignment in Nia

Body awareness is a cornerstone of the Nia Technique, emphasizing mindfulness and presence during movement.

Nia practitioners cultivate a deep connection with their bodies, tuning into sensations, posture, and alignment. Through conscious movement exploration, practitioners enhance their proprioception—the awareness of their body's position in space—and kinesthetic intelligence.

Alignment in Nia refers to the optimal positioning of the body during exercises and routines. Practitioners learn about posture alignment principles that promote balance, stability, and efficient movement mechanics.

This includes aligning the spine, hips, shoulders, and limbs in a way that minimizes strain and maximizes effectiveness.

Nia's approach to body awareness and alignment involves gentle cues and imagery to guide practitioners into proper form and technique.

Practitioners are encouraged to listen to their bodies, make adjustments as needed, and move in a way that feels natural and comfortable.

This focus on alignment not only enhances the aesthetic quality of movements but also reduces the risk of injuries and supports long-term physical well-being.

Nia's Approach to Flexibility and Strength

Flexibility and strength are integrated seamlessly into the Nia Technique, promoting a balanced and harmonious approach to fitness.

Nia recognizes the importance of both qualities in enhancing overall mobility, resilience, and vitality. Through dynamic movements and mindful stretching, practitioners develop flexibility that supports fluidity and ease of movement.

Nia's approach to flexibility goes beyond traditional static stretching, incorporating dynamic stretches, spiraling movements, and rhythmic patterns. This dynamic flexibility training improves joint mobility, muscle elasticity, and range of motion, enhancing functional movement capabilities in daily life.

Strength training in Nia focuses on functional strength—the ability to perform daily tasks with efficiency and ease.

Practitioners engage in body-weight exercises, resistance training with props like hand weights or resistance bands, and functional movements that mimic real-life activities.

This holistic approach to strength development not only builds muscular endurance and tone but also improves posture, stability, and coordination.

By blending flexibility and strength training, Nia practitioners achieve a balanced and adaptable physical condition that supports their overall well-being and enhances their movement quality.

Breathing Techniques in Nia

Breath is a vital component of the Nia Technique, serving as a bridge between mind, body, and spirit. Nia practitioners explore various breathing techniques that facilitate relaxation, energy flow, and mindfulness during movement.

Conscious breathing not only enhances the effectiveness of physical exercises but also promotes mental clarity and emotional balance.

In Nia, practitioners are guided to synchronize their breath with movement, creating a harmonious rhythm that promotes flow and continuity.

Deep diaphragmatic breathing is emphasized, allowing for full oxygenation of the body and a sense of grounding and centering.

Practitioners learn to use breath awareness as a tool for managing stress, releasing tension, and cultivating presence in the moment.

Nia's approach to breathing techniques extends beyond the physical benefits, incorporating elements of meditation and mindfulness.

Practitioners engage in breath-focused practices that quiet the mind, enhance body awareness, and foster a deeper connection with the self.

This mindful breathing practice in Nia serves as a foundation for holistic well-being, integrating the body's physiological responses with mental and emotional states.

CHAPTER 4
Getting Started With Nia

Getting Started with Nia can be an exciting journey into the world of mindful movement and holistic fitness. Whether you're a seasoned fitness enthusiast looking to expand your repertoire or a beginner curious about exploring new avenues of wellness, Nia offers a unique blend of dance, martial arts, and healing arts that can transform your physical and mental well-being.

In this exploration of Getting Started with Nia, we'll delve into essential aspects such as preparing for your first Nia class, setting up your practice space, choosing appropriate clothing and footwear, and crucial safety considerations and injury prevention strategies.

Preparing for Your First Nia Class involves several key steps to ensure a fulfilling and enjoyable experience. First and foremost, familiarize yourself with the philosophy and principles of Nia.

Understanding that Nia is not just about physical exercise but also about self-expression, joy, and mindfulness sets the right tone for your practice. It's also beneficial to research and choose a certified Nia instructor or studio that aligns with your goals and preferences. Communicate any health concerns or physical limitations to your instructor beforehand to receive personalized guidance and modifications during the class.

Setting Up Your Practice Space plays a significant role in creating a conducive environment for Nia's practice. Ideally, choose a space that is free from clutter and distractions, allowing you to move freely and connect with your body.

Ensure adequate lighting and ventilation to enhance your comfort and focus. Consider adding elements like calming music, candles, or essential oils to create a soothing atmosphere that enhances your mind-body connection during Nia sessions.

Choosing Appropriate Clothing and Footwear for Nia is essential for unrestricted movement and comfort. Opt for breathable, moisture-wicking fabrics that allow your skin to breathe and move effortlessly. Loose-fitting clothing that doesn't restrict your range of motion is ideal for Nia's dynamic movements. When it comes to footwear, many Nia practitioners prefer to go barefoot or wear minimalistic shoes that provide grip and support without compromising flexibility.

Safety Considerations and Injury Prevention are paramount in any fitness practice, including Nia. Start slowly and listen to your body's signals during each movement.

Avoid pushing yourself beyond your limits and honor your body's needs for rest and recovery. Warm up before each session to prepare your muscles and joints for movement, and incorporate gradual progressions to avoid strain or injury.

If you have any pre-existing medical conditions or injuries, consult with your healthcare provider before engaging in Nia or any new fitness regimen.

By taking proactive steps in preparing for your Nia journey, including understanding the fundamentals, setting up an inviting practice space, choosing suitable attire and footwear, and prioritizing safety and injury prevention, you set yourself up for a rewarding and sustainable experience with Nia's transformative practices.

CHAPTER 5
Nia Technique For Fitness And Wellness

Nia Technique, a fusion of dance, martial arts, and healing arts, offers a unique approach to fitness and wellness. This holistic practice not only enhances physical fitness but also promotes mental and emotional well-being.

In this exploration, we delve into the various facets of Nia for beginners, focusing on its contributions to cardiovascular health, strength and conditioning, stress reduction, relaxation, mindfulness, and emotional well-being.

Nia for Cardiovascular Health

Cardiovascular health is a cornerstone of overall well-being, and Nia offers a dynamic pathway to enhance this aspect of fitness. Through its rhythmic movements, Nia stimulates cardiovascular endurance, promoting efficient heart function and circulation.

The incorporation of dance elements in Nia sessions elevates heart rate variability, a key indicator of cardiovascular fitness. Furthermore, the diversity of movements in Nia, from flowing to percussive, engages different muscle groups, supporting cardiovascular conditioning across the body. Regular participation in Nia can lead to improved cardiovascular endurance, reduced risk of heart disease, and increased stamina for daily activities.

Strength and Conditioning with Nia

While often associated with graceful movements, Nia is also a potent tool for strength and conditioning. The integration of martial arts-inspired techniques brings elements of strength training into Nia sessions.

Movements such as punches, kicks, and blocks activate muscles throughout the body, fostering muscular strength and endurance. Additionally, Nia emphasizes functional movement patterns that mimic real-life activities, enhancing overall physical capabilities.

Through consistent practice, individuals can experience enhanced muscular tone, improved posture, and increased resilience against injuries.

Nia's Role in Stress Reduction and Relaxation

In today's fast-paced world, stress management is paramount for holistic well-being. Nia provides a sanctuary for stress reduction and relaxation through its mindful approach to movement.

The incorporation of breath awareness and conscious movement allows participants to enter a state of deep relaxation during Nia sessions.

The rhythmic flow of movements coupled with uplifting music creates a meditative environment, promoting relaxation of both body and mind. Regular practice of Nia can lead to reduced stress levels, improved sleep quality, and a greater sense of inner calm and balance.

Nia for Mindfulness and Emotional Well-being

Mindfulness, the practice of being present in the moment, is a central theme in Nia. Through mindful movement and body awareness, Nia cultivates a deeper connection between the mind and body.

Participants are encouraged to explore sensations, emotions, and thoughts that arise during movement, fostering self-awareness and emotional intelligence.

The expressive nature of Nia allows individuals to release pent-up emotions and channel positive energy through movement. This integration of mindfulness and emotional expression promotes mental clarity, emotional resilience, and overall well-being.

the Nia Technique for beginners offers a multifaceted approach to fitness and wellness, encompassing cardiovascular health, strength and conditioning, stress reduction, relaxation, mindfulness, and emotional well-being.

Through its diverse movements, mindful practices, and holistic philosophy, Nia empowers individuals to cultivate a harmonious balance between physical vitality and inner peace.

CHAPTER 6
Exploring Nia Routines And Choreography

Introduction to Nia Routines: Nia routines form the foundation of the Nia practice, providing a structured framework within which practitioners can explore movement, express themselves, and connect with their bodies and emotions.

These routines are meticulously designed to incorporate a blend of movements from various disciplines, including jazz dance, modern dance, tai chi, aikido, and yoga. The diversity of movement styles ensures a comprehensive workout that targets flexibility, strength, balance, agility, and cardiovascular endurance.

Within Nia routines, practitioners encounter a rhythmic flow that seamlessly transitions between slow, mindful movements and dynamic, expressive sequences. This rhythmic variation not only challenges the body but also engages the mind, fostering a sense of mindfulness and presence during the practice. Each routine is thoughtfully crafted to synchronize breath with movement, enhancing body awareness and promoting a deeper mind-body connection.

Creating Flow and Harmony in Movement Sequences: Central to the Nia experience is the concept of flow—a state of effortless movement characterized by smooth transitions, fluidity, and grace.

Creating flow within movement sequences involves a harmonious integration of different body parts, rhythmic patterns, and spatial awareness. Practitioners are encouraged to explore the natural flow of their bodies, allowing movements to unfold organically and expressively.

Key elements that contribute to flow in Nia include:

1. Breath Awareness: Conscious breathing patterns guide the pace and rhythm of movements, facilitating a seamless flow between poses and transitions.

2. Dynamic Range of Motion: Embracing the full range of motion in joints and muscles adds fluidity and grace to movements, avoiding stiffness or rigidity.

3. Emotional Expression: Infusing movements with emotion and intention brings authenticity and depth to the practice, creating a dynamic interplay between physical and emotional states.

4. Spatial Awareness: Being mindful of spatial dynamics, such as levels (high, middle, low), pathways (linear, circular), and directions (forward, backward, sideways), enhances movement quality and flow.

By cultivating flow and harmony in movement sequences, practitioners not only enhance the aesthetic appeal of their dance but also experience a sense of freedom, creativity, and self-expression.

Choreographing Your Nia Dance: One of the unique aspects of Nia is the opportunity for practitioners to choreograph their dances within the framework of Nia principles and techniques. Choreography in Nia is a creative process that encourages individual expression, personal style, and exploration of movement possibilities.

When choreographing a Nia dance, practitioners can follow these steps:

1. Inspiration: Begin by finding inspiration from music, emotions, themes, or personal experiences. Allow your creativity to flow freely without judgment.

2. Movement Exploration: Experiment with different movements, gestures, poses, and sequences that resonate with your body and intentions. Focus on fluid transitions and rhythmic variations.

3. Structure: Organize your movements into coherent sequences or patterns, considering elements such as tempo changes, directional shifts, and emotional dynamics.

4. Music Selection: Choose music that complements your choreography and enhances the mood and energy of your dance. Pay attention to musical cues for timing and synchronization.

5. Practice and Refinement: Rehearse your choreography regularly, refining movements, transitions, and timing. Invite feedback from peers or instructors to improve your dance.

Choreographing your own Nia dance allows for personalization and creative expression, empowering practitioners to embody their unique artistic vision and storytelling through movement.

Nia Music and its Influence on Movement: Music plays a pivotal role in the Nia experience, catalyzing movement, emotion, and energy.

The selection of music in Nia is diverse, encompassing genres such as world music, pop, jazz, ambient, and tribal beats.

Each piece of music contributes to the atmosphere, mood, and rhythm of the Nia practice, influencing the pace, intensity, and style of movement.

The influence of Nia music on movement can be observed through several aspects:

1. Rhythm and Tempo: The rhythmic patterns and tempo of music inspire specific movement qualities, such as flowing, staccato, chaos, lyrical, and stillness.

Practitioners synchronize their movements with the beat and energy of the music, creating a dynamic and engaging dance experience.

2. Emotional Resonance: Music evokes emotions and feelings that are translated into movement expressions. Slow, melodic tunes may invite

introspection and fluidity, while upbeat rhythms can stimulate energy and playfulness.

3. Creativity and Interpretation: The interpretation of music is highly individualized, allowing practitioners to interpret lyrics, melodies, and rhythms in their unique ways. This freedom of interpretation fuels creativity and improvisation in movement.

4. Energy Management: Music acts as an energy regulator, guiding the intensity and pacing of the practice.

Transitions between high-energy tracks and calming melodies contribute to a balanced and holistic movement experience.

In Nia, practitioners develop a symbiotic relationship with music, allowing it to guide, inspire, and elevate their movement journey.

The fusion of music and movement creates a transformative experience that nurtures body, mind, and spirit.

By exploring Nia's routines and choreography, practitioners unlock a world of movement possibilities, creativity, and self-expression. Through flow, harmony, choreographic exploration, and musical integration, Nia becomes not just a fitness practice but a holistic journey of embodiment, artistry, and joyous movement.

CHAPTER 7
Adapting Nia For Different Needs

Nia, a fusion fitness practice blending dance, martial arts, and healing arts, offers a versatile platform adaptable to various age groups and physical conditions. Understanding the principles of adapting Nia for different needs involves a nuanced approach that respects individual capabilities while maximizing the benefits of movement and mindfulness.

Nia for All Ages: Children, Adults, Seniors

Incorporating Nia into the lives of individuals across all age groups presents unique opportunities and considerations. For children, Nia can be a joyful introduction to movement, fostering creativity, coordination, and body awareness. Structured classes can incorporate storytelling, music, and playful movements that resonate with young learners. Adults engaging in Nia experience a holistic workout that addresses physical fitness, stress relief, and self-expression. The adaptable nature of Nia allows adults to tailor their practice to their fitness levels, whether they seek a vigorous cardio workout or a gentle mind-body session. Seniors benefit significantly from Nia's gentle approach, promoting flexibility, balance, and emotional well-being. Modifications and mindful movements cater to the needs of older adults, ensuring a safe and enjoyable experience.

Nia Modifications for Physical Limitations

One of Nia's strengths lies in its adaptability to individuals with physical limitations. Whether due to injury, chronic conditions, or temporary setbacks, Nia offers modifications that allow participants to engage in meaningful movement without compromising safety. For example, individuals with joint issues can adjust movements to reduce impact, focusing on range of motion and fluidity. Those with mobility challenges can explore seated variations or use supportive props to maintain participation and benefit from the practice. Nia instructors trained in modification techniques play a crucial role in ensuring inclusivity and accessibility for all participants.

Nia for Rehabilitation and Recovery

The therapeutic potential of Nia extends to rehabilitation and recovery settings, where movement becomes a tool for healing and restoration. Integrating Nia into rehabilitation programs for injuries or surgeries offers a holistic approach to recovery, addressing physical, emotional, and psychological aspects. The mindful nature of Nia promotes body awareness, aiding in relearning movement patterns and rebuilding strength. In recovery from trauma or illness, Nia's gentle movements and focus on breath can support individuals in reconnecting with their bodies and fostering a sense of well-being.

Nia in Special Populations: Pregnancy, Postpartum, Disabilities

Special populations, including pregnant individuals, postpartum mothers, and those with disabilities, can benefit from tailored Nia practices designed to meet their specific needs. Pregnancy-focused Nia classes emphasize gentle movements, pelvic floor awareness, and breathing techniques that support maternal health and well-being. Postpartum Nia offers a gradual return to movement, addressing core strength, posture, and emotional balance during the recovery period. For individuals with disabilities, Nia instructors collaborate with healthcare professionals to create adaptive programs that prioritize safety, inclusion, and empowerment through movement.

Overall, adapting Nia to different needs requires a compassionate approach rooted in understanding individual capabilities and goals. By embracing modifications, specialized programs, and inclusive practices, Nia continues to serve as a transformative and inclusive movement practice for all.

CHAPTER 8
Integrating Nia Into Daily Life

Integrating Nia into daily life involves more than just practicing the movements in a studio setting; it's about embodying the principles and mindset of Nia in various aspects of one's routine. By understanding how to apply Nia outside of dance sessions, individuals can enhance their well-being, manage stress effectively, and cultivate a more mindful approach to everyday activities.

Incorporating Nia principles off the dance floor requires a conscious effort to integrate the core concepts of Nia into daily routines. This includes embodying the three core principles of Nia—Dance, Martial Arts, and Healing Arts—in simple tasks such as walking, sitting, or even standing.

By focusing on the sensation of movement and the connection between body, mind, and spirit, individuals can experience a sense of mindfulness and presence in their actions.

Nia for stress management at work offers a unique approach to dealing with daily pressures and challenges. By incorporating Nia movements, breathing techniques, and mindful awareness into work breaks or desk routines, individuals can reduce stress levels, improve focus and concentration, and enhance overall well-being. The rhythmic and flowing movements of Nia can help release tension, increase energy levels, and promote a sense of calmness amidst a busy work environment.

Using Nia movements in everyday activities involves incorporating Nia-inspired techniques into common tasks such as cooking, cleaning, or gardening. By infusing these movements with intention, grace, and awareness, individuals can turn mundane activities into mindful practices that promote physical fitness, flexibility, and body awareness. This integration of Nia into daily life fosters a holistic approach to health and wellness, where movement becomes a source of joy and self-expression.

Cultivating a Nia mindset beyond the studio extends beyond physical movements; it encompasses a mindset of self-care, self-expression, and self-discovery.

By adopting Nia's philosophy of pleasure, playfulness, and mindfulness, individuals can navigate life's challenges with resilience, creativity, and authenticity. This mindset encourages a balanced lifestyle, where movement, rest, and reflection are valued equally, leading to greater overall well-being and fulfillment.

Integrating Nia into daily life goes beyond dance routines; it's about embracing a holistic approach to health, wellness, and personal growth.

By incorporating Nia principles, movements, and mindset into everyday activities, individuals can experience a profound transformation in how they move, think, and live.

CHAPTER 9
Nia Community And Resources

The Nia community is a vibrant and supportive network of individuals who share a passion for holistic fitness and mindful movement.

Within this community, practitioners find not only physical health benefits but also a sense of belonging and connection. Understanding the resources available within the Nia community is crucial for beginners embarking on their journey into this unique movement practice.

Finding Nia Classes and Certified Instructors

One of the first steps for beginners interested in Nia is finding classes and instructors who are certified in the Nia technique. Nia classes are typically offered in fitness centers, yoga studios, community centers, and online platforms. The Nia Technique website provides a comprehensive directory of certified instructors and Nia classes worldwide, making it easy for newcomers to locate classes in their area or online.

Certified Nia instructors undergo rigorous training to teach the Nia technique effectively. They blend dance, martial arts, and healing arts seamlessly, creating a holistic movement experience for participants. Beginners benefit from the expertise and guidance of certified instructors who can introduce them to Nia's principles and help them develop proper form and technique.

Joining Nia Communities and Events

Joining Nia communities and attending events is an enriching experience for beginners. Nia communities often organize workshops, retreats, and special events that delve deeper into the practice and offer opportunities for personal growth. These gatherings bring together like-minded individuals who are passionate about health, wellness, and self-expression through movement.

Online forums and social media groups also serve as virtual communities where Nia practitioners can connect, share experiences, ask questions, and support each other on their Nia journey. Engaging with these communities fosters a sense of camaraderie and encourages ongoing learning and exploration.

Nia Books, Videos, and Online Resources

For beginners seeking to deepen their understanding of Nia beyond the studio, a wealth of resources is available. Nia books written by founder Debbie Rosas and other experienced instructors offer insights into the philosophy, techniques, and benefits of Nia. These books often include illustrated guides to Nia movements, mindfulness practices, and holistic wellness tips.

Videos and online classes allow beginners to practice Nia at home or while traveling, providing flexibility and convenience. Online platforms like NiaTV offer a library of classes for all levels, including specialized sessions for beginners, intermediate practitioners, and advanced students. These resources empower beginners to continue their Nia practice outside of structured classes and explore different styles and instructors.

Testimonials and Success Stories from Nia Practitioners

Reading testimonials and success stories from fellow Nia practitioners can be inspiring and motivating for beginners. Real-life experiences shared by individuals who have benefited from Nia's transformative effects highlight its impact on physical fitness, mental well-being, and overall quality of life. These stories often emphasize increased energy, reduced stress, improved body awareness, and enhanced self-confidence.

Testimonials also provide insights into the diverse ways people incorporate Nia into their lives, whether as a daily practice, a supplement to other fitness routines, or a means of artistic expression. Beginners can gain valuable perspective and encouragement from these narratives, reinforcing their commitment to exploring and embracing the Nia technique.

By engaging with the Nia community and utilizing available resources, beginners can embark on a fulfilling journey of self-discovery, holistic wellness, and joyful movement through the Nia technique.

CHAPTER 10
Nia For Long-Term Wellness

Nia, a holistic movement practice blending dance, martial arts, and healing arts, offers profound benefits for long-term wellness. At its core, Nia promotes a balanced integration of body, mind, emotions, and spirit, making it a versatile and sustainable approach to overall well-being.

Unlike traditional fitness routines focused solely on physical outcomes, Nia emphasizes self-expression, joy in movement, and self-awareness, fostering a deeper connection with oneself and the surrounding environment.

Central to Nia's philosophy is the concept of pleasure in movement. By prioritizing enjoyment and sensation in every motion, practitioners develop a positive relationship with exercise, making it more likely to be embraced as a lifelong practice. This emphasis on pleasure also encourages individuals to listen to their bodies, honoring their unique needs and limitations, thus reducing the risk of burnout or injury commonly associated with rigid exercise regimens.

One of the key aspects of Nia's long-term wellness benefits is its adaptability to different fitness levels and life stages. Whether someone is a beginner just starting their fitness journey or a seasoned athlete seeking new challenges, Nia offers a variety of movement options and modifications to suit individual capabilities and goals. This inclusivity not only makes Nia accessible to a wide range of people but also fosters a sense of community and support within Nia classes or groups.

Setting Goals and Tracking Progress in Nia

Setting clear and achievable goals is fundamental to progress and motivation in any fitness practice, including Nia. When beginning a Nia journey, it's essential to identify personal objectives, whether they involve improving physical fitness, enhancing body awareness, reducing stress, or simply finding joy in movement. These goals serve as guiding lights, keeping practitioners focused and motivated during their Nia practice.

In Nia, goal setting goes beyond mere physical accomplishments; it encompasses emotional, mental, and spiritual aspirations as well.

For instance, a goal might involve cultivating a greater sense of self-confidence, exploring creativity through movement, or deepening mindfulness and presence during workouts.

By embracing a holistic approach to goal setting, individuals can experience profound transformations that extend far beyond the physical realm.

Tracking progress in Nia involves more than just measuring tangible outcomes like weight loss or muscle strength. It includes observing subtle shifts in energy levels, emotional resilience, and overall well-being. Practitioners may keep journals to note their experiences, insights, and reflections after each Nia session, allowing them to track their growth and celebrate milestones along the way.

Creating a Sustainable Nia Practice Routine

Sustainability is a cornerstone of Nia's approach to fitness and wellness. Unlike fad diets or extreme workout programs that often lead to burnout or unsustainable results, Nia encourages a balanced and mindful approach to movement that can be sustained over the long term. Creating a sustainable Nia practice routine involves several key elements:

1. Variety and Adaptability: Nia offers a diverse range of movements, from gentle stretches to dynamic cardio sequences, ensuring that practitioners can adapt their practice to their current energy levels, physical abilities, and mood. This variety prevents monotony and keeps the practice fresh and engaging.

2. Rest and Recovery: Nia recognizes the importance of rest and recovery in promoting overall well-being. Practitioners are encouraged to listen to their bodies and incorporate rest days or gentle movement practices, such as Nia's "Liquid Motion," to support recovery and prevent overtraining.

3. Mindful Movement: Mindfulness is integral to sustainable fitness practices. Nia teaches practitioners to pay attention to their bodies' signals, such as sensations of tension or fatigue, and adjust their movement accordingly. This mindful approach reduces the risk of injury and supports longevity in practice.

4. Community and Support: Building a community of fellow Nia practitioners can enhance motivation and accountability. Group classes or online communities provide opportunities for connection, encouragement, and shared experiences, fostering a sense of belonging and support.

5. Integration into Daily Life: Nia is not just a workout; it's a way of life. Practitioners are encouraged to integrate Nia principles, such as mindfulness, pleasure in movement, and self-expression, into their daily activities. This integration ensures that the benefits of Nia extend beyond the studio into all aspects of life.

Celebrating Milestones and Achievements

Celebrating milestones and achievements is an essential part of maintaining motivation and enthusiasm in a Nia practice. Whether it's mastering a new movement pattern, completing a series of classes, or experiencing a breakthrough in self-awareness, each achievement deserves recognition and celebration. Here are some ways to celebrate milestones in Nia:

1. Acknowledge Progress: Take time to acknowledge and appreciate the progress you've made, no matter how small.

Reflect on the changes you've noticed in your body, mind, and spirit since starting your Nia practice.

2. Set Rewards: Establish rewards for reaching specific milestones or goals. These rewards can be non-material, such as scheduling a self-care day or treating yourself to a relaxing activity, or they can be tangible rewards that motivate you to keep pushing forward.

3. Share Successes: Share your successes with your Nia community or supportive friends and family. Celebrating achievements with others not only amplifies the joy but also inspires and motivates fellow practitioners on their journeys.

4. Create Rituals: Develop rituals or traditions around milestone celebrations. This could involve a special movement sequence, a gratitude practice, or a symbolic gesture that marks your achievements and reinforces your commitment to continued growth.

By celebrating milestones and achievements in Nia, practitioners cultivate a positive mindset, boost their self-confidence, and stay inspired to pursue their wellness goals with passion and dedication.

Nia's Role in Lifelong Fitness and Well-being

Nia's holistic approach to movement and wellness positions it as a valuable tool for lifelong fitness and well-being. Unlike traditional exercise programs that focus solely on physical fitness or aesthetics, Nia addresses the interconnectedness of body, mind, emotions, and spirit, promoting a comprehensive and sustainable approach to health.

One of Nia's strengths in supporting lifelong fitness is its adaptability to changing needs and abilities. As individuals progress through different life stages, from youth to middle age to senior years, Nia offers a flexible framework that can be modified to accommodate varying energy levels, mobility challenges, and health considerations. This adaptability ensures that Nia remains relevant and beneficial throughout one's entire life.

Furthermore, Nia's emphasis on pleasure in movement and self-expression makes it an enjoyable and fulfilling practice that individuals are more likely to stick with over the long term. The joy and satisfaction experienced during Nia workouts contribute to mental and emotional well-being, reducing stress, enhancing mood, and fostering a positive relationship with exercise.

Nia also plays a crucial role in promoting functional fitness, which focuses on improving everyday movements and activities.

By incorporating functional movement patterns into Nia routines, practitioners develop strength, flexibility, balance, and coordination that directly translate to enhanced quality of life and independence.

In essence, Nia's holistic approach, adaptability, emphasis on pleasure, and focus on functional fitness make it a valuable companion in the journey toward lifelong fitness and well-being.

By embracing Nia as more than just a workout but as a lifestyle that nurtures body, mind, and spirit, individuals can experience lasting health benefits and a deeper connection to themselves and the world around them.

Conclusion

In the vibrant world of Nia Technique for Beginners, you've embarked on a journey that intertwines movement, mindfulness, and holistic wellness. Discovering the essence of Nia has unveiled a tapestry of sensations, from the rhythmic dance steps to the grounding techniques of martial arts and the soothing embrace of healing arts. Here, you've found not just a workout but a way of life that celebrates your body's innate wisdom and joy in movement.

Your exploration into Nia's rich tapestry of movements, encompassing dance, martial arts, and healing arts principles, has been a revelation of self-discovery. Embodying each of the 52 Nia Moves has been a dance of sensation and pleasure, where the mind-body connection blooms into a harmonious symphony of wellness.

Delving into the anatomy of Nia, you've honed your body awareness and alignment, embracing flexibility, strength, and the rhythm of breath as allies in your practice. Every step, every stretch, and every breath has become a testament to your journey towards holistic well-being.

As you ventured into your first Nia class, the preparations, safety considerations, and the choice of attire became not just rituals but gateways to a transformative experience. Nia's fusion of cardiovascular health, strength conditioning, stress reduction, and mindfulness has woven a fabric of vitality and resilience in your life.

Exploring Nia's diverse routines and choreography has not only unleashed your creativity but also deepened your connection with movement. Adapting Nia to different needs, from children to seniors, and its role in rehabilitation and special populations has broadened your understanding of inclusivity and adaptability in fitness.

Integrating Nia into your daily life has been a revelation of mindful living beyond the studio. From stress management at work to infusing Nia principles into everyday activities, you've cultivated a Nia mindset that transcends the dance floor, enriching every moment with presence and purpose.

Embracing the Nia community, resources, and testimonials has woven a tapestry of support and inspiration, fueling your commitment to long-term wellness. Setting goals, tracking progress, and celebrating milestones have become not just rituals but affirmations of your dedication to lifelong fitness and well-being.

your journey through the Nia Technique for Beginners, remember that every step you've taken, every move you've embodied, and every moment of joy and self-discovery has been a celebration of your true essence. Nia isn't just about movement; it's about embracing life with vitality, grace, and an unwavering commitment to your holistic wellness journey.

www.ingramcontent.com/pod-product-compliance
Lightning Source LLC
Chambersburg PA
CBHW051703250726
48653CB00007B/2816